Gastric Bypass Recipes

80+ Simple Recipes for the First Stage After Gastric Bypass

John Carter

Table of Contents

Bonus: FREE Report Reveals The Secrets To Lose Weight

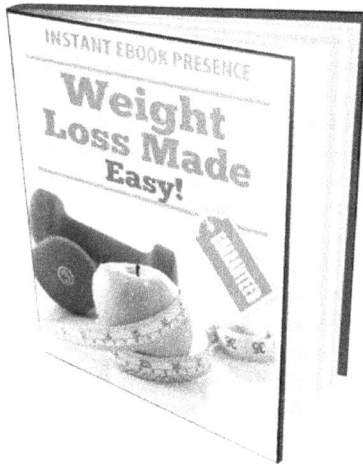

Weight loss doesn't happen from dieting only. Diets are short term solutions to shed extra weight. Diets do not work in the long term because people hate being on a diet (it's ok, you can admit that here). The only long term solution for permanent weight loss is to create new eating habits. This doesn't mean that chocolate will never pass your lips again, but it does mean looking after yourself and watching what you eat...

You can lose weight when you have the right reasons and motivation, and a part of this guide is to help you to find the motivation you need to change your weight...

Introduction

Congratulations on downloading your personal copy of *Gastric Bypass Recipes*. Thank you for doing so.

The following chapters will provide you with information to help you through the first stages after you have your gastric bypass surgery

You will discover how important it is to control what and how you eat so that you don't experience any adverse effects.

There are plenty of books on this subject on the market, thanks again for choosing this one! Every effort was made to ensure it is full of as much useful information as possible. Please enjoy!

Congratulations on downloading your personal copy of *Gastric Bypass Recipes*. Thank you for doing so.

Guide for the After Surgery

People who have undergone gastric bypass surgery will have to follow a specific diet, especially right after their operation. They will gradually learn how to they can and can't eat so that they don't experience any discomfort.

Gastric bypass is only one form of weight-loss surgeries that are currently performed. The operation has undergone many changes since it was first used. The gastric bypass that is performed today is known as Roux-en-Y. Do not confuse gastric bypass with other weight-loss operations such as biliopancreatic diversion with duodenal switch as this kind of surgery is a lot more aggressive. When you have the surgery, you will talk with your dietitian or doctor, and they will inform on how you should eat after your operation, and they will explain the foods that can eat and how much. If you follow the plan they out for you closely, then you will safely lose weight.

To help get you started, and in the right mindset, let's look at what your doctor is likely to tell you.

There are many reasons why a person starts following a gastric bypass diet. These include:

- To keep from experiencing complications or side effect after the surgery

- To avoid gaining weight and to help them lose weight

- To help you become used to eating smaller portions of food that your stomach will be able to safely and comfortably digest

- To give the stomach time to heal so that the food you eat won't stretch it out

The diet recommendations that you receive after surgery typically vary depending on who does your surgery, where you get it done, and your situation. You will first go through different stages right after your surgery before you enter into your gastric bypass diet. The movement through these stages will depend on how well you heal and can adjust to the new eating patterns. You will likely be able to eat regular foods three months after the surgery.

After you have your surgery, you have to make sure that you drink plenty of fluids so that you don't become dehydrated, and to pay attention to when you feel full or hungry.

On the first day or two after your surgery, you will only get to drink clear liquids. You will have to sip slowly, and you can only drink two to three ounces at a time. After you can handle clear liquids, you will be able to start having other types of liquids, like low-fat or skim milk.

During stage one you can have:

- Sugar-free popsicles or gelatin
- Strained cream soup
- 1% or skim milk
- Decaf coffee or tea
- Unsweetened juice broth

After your system has become used to only liquids for a couple of days, you can start eating pureed and strained foods. You should only consume foods that are the consistency of a thick liquid or smooth paste, without the presence of solid pieces in the mix.

When you are picking foods to puree it best to pick foods that blend well, like:

- Cottage cheese
- Cooked vegetables and soft fruits
- Eggs
- Fish
- Beans
- Lean ground meats

Use these liquids to blend with:

- Broth
- No sugar added juice
- Skim milk
- Water

It's also important to remember that you shouldn't drink and eat at the same time. You need to wait 30 minutes after you eat before you drink anything. Keep in mind that during this time that your digestive system can still be sensitive to certain foods like dairy or spicy foods. If you want to start eating these foods at this time, slowly add them back into your diet with small amounts.

Once you receive your doctor's okay, after a few weeks on pureed foods, you can start to add in soft foods. These should be in the form of tender, small, and easily chewed pieces. During this time, you can start adding:

- Cooked vegetables, without the skin
- Canned or soft fresh fruit, with the seeds and skin, removed
- Finely diced or ground meats

After you have been on this diet for about eight weeks, you will be able to slowly add in firmer foods, but you need to make sure that they are diced or chopped. Make sure you slowly add in regular foods to find out what you can tolerate. You may discover that you still have a hard time with spicy foods, or with foods that have a crunchy texture.

Even once you reach this stage, there are certain foods that you shouldn't eat because they can cause symptoms like vomiting, nausea, or pain. You should avoid:

- Breads
- Fried foods
- Meats with gristle or tough meats
- Fibrous or stringy vegetables, like cabbage, corn, broccoli, or celery
- Granola
- Carbonated beverages
- Dried fruits
- Popcorn
- Seeds and nuts

After some time, you can try to add these foods back into your diet with your doctor's guidance.

Once you hit three to four months after your surgery, you will be able to begin eating a healthy and normal diet, depending on what your situation is, and depending on the foods that you can't tolerate. It's also possible that foods you found irritating right after your surgery, you can now eat after you stomach has healed.

To make sure that you receive enough minerals and vitamins, and to keep yourself on track for your weight-loss goals, at every stage of your diet, make sure you:

- Drink and eat slowly. When you eat or drink too fast, you may experience dumping syndrome. This is when liquids and foods enter into your small intestine quickly and in a larger amount than normal, which causes sweating, dizziness, vomiting, nausea, and soon, diarrhea. To prevent this from happening, eat liquids and foods low in sugar and fat, drink and eat slowly, and then wait 30 to 45 minutes after every meal to drink. Eating your meal should take at least 30 minutes, and it should take 30 to 60 minutes to drink a cup of liquid.

- Eat small meals. As your diet progresses, you should eat many small meals throughout the day, and slowly sip liquids. You may even want to start with six small meals a day at first, move towards four meals, and then return to a regular diet of three meals each day. Every meal should have a half-cup to a cup of food. You should only eat the recommended serving, and make sure to stop eating before you are full.

- Have your liquids between meals. You should drink six to eight cups of fluids each day so that you don't become dehydrated. If you drink liquids with your meals, you will likely feel pain, nausea, and sometimes vomiting, along with the dumping syndrome. If you drink too much around the time of your meal, you may feel too full and can prevent you from eating foods that are nutrient-rich.

- Thoroughly chew your food. The opening that the surgeon created that leads from the stomach to the intestine is tiny, and big pieces of foods may block this opening. Blockages will prevent food from leaving the stomach and will lead to abdominal pain, vomiting, and nausea. Eat small bites, and completely chew them before you swallow. If you are unable to thoroughly chew the food, then do not swallow it.

- Eat foods high in protein. Right after your surgery, eating high-protein foods will help you to heal. Low-fat, high-protein choices should stay as a good long-term diet choice after surgery. Add in lean cuts of beans, fish, pork, chicken, or beef. Low-fat yogurts, cottage cheese, and cheese are also good sources of protein.

- Keep away from foods that are high in sugar and fat. After you have your surgery, it can be hard on the digestive system to tolerate foods that contain a lot of sugars and fat. Keep away from foods like candy bars, fried foods, and ice cream because they are high in fat. Choose sugar-free options like dairy products and soft drinks.

- Introduce foods one at a time. There will be certain foods that you eat after surgery that can cause vomiting, pain, nausea, or can block the opening to your stomach. It will vary from person to person as to what foods they will be able to tolerate. Add new foods one at a time, and make sure you completely chew it. If what you eat causes any discomfort, don't continue to eat it. As more time passes, you may find that you can eat it. Liquids and foods that tend to cause discomfort are carbonated beverages, fried foods, raw veggies, bread, and meat.

- Take mineral vitamin supplements. Since a part of your small intestine will be bypassed after surgery, the body will have problems absorbing the need nutrients from your food. You will probably have to take a multivitamin every day for the remainder of your life. You will need to talk with your doctor as to which vitamin is best for you and if there is any need for you to take anything else, like calcium.

Long term weight loss will be the likely result from your gastric bypass surgery. How much you lose will depend on the kind of weight-loss surgery you have and the lifestyle changes that you make. It is even likely that you will be able to lose half, or more, of the excess weight that you need to within two years time.

This diet will help you to recover from your surgery and to transition into a healthy eating routine and to support your goals for weight-loss. If you return to your old unhealthy eating habits after your surgery, you will probably not lose the weight you need to, or you could gain weight back that you have lost.

The biggest problems that you can encounter from a gastric bypass diet come from not following it properly. When you eat too much or consume foods that you shouldn't, you may experience complications. Complications could include:

- Dumping syndrome. This will typically happen if you eat foods that are high in fat or sugar. These foods have a tendency to travel fast through the stomach pouch and will dump into the intestine. When you experience dumping syndrome, it is accompanied by sweating, dizziness, vomiting, nausea, and diarrhea.

- Dehydration. Since you can't drink fluids along with your meals, people may experience dehydration. To prevent the dehydration, you should sip on 48 to 64 ounces of water each day and other types of low-calorie drinks.

- Vomiting and nausea. When you eat too fast, too much, or don't thoroughly chew your food, you may experience vomiting and nausea after your meals.

- Constipation. When you don't keep a regular eating schedule, don't consume enough fiber, or you don't exercise, you might end up becoming constipated.

- Stomach pouch opening becomes blocked. It's completely possible that food becomes lodged in the opening of your stomach, even if you are extremely careful about following your diet. Symptoms of having a blocked stomach are an abdominal pain, nausea, and vomiting. If you suffer from these symptoms for more than a couple of days, call your doctor.

- Failure to lose weight or weight gain. If you start to gain weight after your surgery, or you don't lose the weight you need to, you may not be eating the right food or consuming too many calories. Speak with your dietitian or doctor to make the best changes for you.

Immediately After Surgery Diet

There are three basic parts of your after surgery diet, no matter which weight-loss surgery you chose to have. In all of them, the first will be fluids, and this will likely be the most challenging. Most people will go home still feeling tired, uncomfortable, and clutching onto their hospital guidelines, and then find themselves wondering in the kitchen unsure of what they should drink or eat.

The first and most important thing is to follow what your bariatric team and surgeon have told you. There will be some surgeons that recommend consuming only clear fluids at first and then adding full fluids during the first few days after surgery; some will have you to continue fluids for a full four weeks after surgery. This is to help minimize digestion, lessen solid waste production, and to ensure maximum healing for the gastrointestinal system.

Clear liquids, the kind you can see through, are the first thing you can start consuming. You should only sip them slowly and never gulp them. You should consume enough so that you stay hydrated, which means you should probably keep a liquid beside you at all times. Make sure that some of these liquids have nutritional qualities so that you receive some nourishment.

Below I will list some of the most common and best choices for liquids, and you will eventually find your favorites. When you first start drinking them, they will likely taste strange, maybe too sweet, so add water or ice to help dilute them so that they have a more acceptable flavor. Variety will likely help during this phase so that you don't end up becoming bored. There may only be a few choices, but it's for the best. These liquids help to maximize your healing process, and you should only move to the next stage when your doctor tells you to.

Generally, you should aim for 2.5 to 3.5 liters of fluid each day. It may seem hard at first to achieve this, but at least try. Spread your drinks out evenly. Everybody will have a different fluid need, and the best way to know if you hydrated is by looking at your urine's color. If your output is pale in color, then you are well hydrated. If it is darker, like straw-colored, or there is only a little bit of urine, you should drink more.

Fluid portion size is recommended to be around six or seven ounces, and in your first few days, this is going to sound like a lot. You should consume each serving about an hour apart. You should also never consume fizzy drinks.

Clear fluid choices include:

- Whey protein isolate fruit drink, such as Syntrax Nectar, mixed with water – this is also good for consuming protein within the early stages

- Vegetable, chicken, or beef broth, bouillon, or consommé, or clear soup
- Sugar-free jelly
- Sugar-free ice pops
- 'Salty' drinks that are diluted in hot water
- Sugar-free or no-sugar-added cordials and squashes
- Coffee, warm and decaffeinated
- Tea, warm and herbal or fruit teas
- Water

It may seem like a long time, but you will eventually move into full liquids, which give you more variety and nutrition. This is an important part because this will prepare your stomach for more solid foods. This stage may last for only a couple of days, or several weeks, it will depend on your surgery and doctor. Follow your surgeon's time line.

Full liquids are the type of foods that are pourable and smooth. Mix and match these liquids with the clear liquids to keep hydrated. The way they taste to you may still be a little strange, so you'll need to experiment, but variety is still important so that you can moves sensibly through this and prepare the body for what's to come. It will get better as each day goes by, and you will develop good habits during this stage and reap those effects better.

Full liquid choices:

- Lightly set egg custards
- Low-sugar and low-fat custards
- Homemade poultry, vegetable, or fish soups, pureed until smooth and then dilute them until they are a runny

consistency. You can gradually increase the thickness as you go on.

- Options or Highlight hot chocolate drinks

- Smooth-type cup-a-soups

- Cocoa – made with skim milk

- Homemade smoothies and store bought ones, make sure they are not thick

- Slimfast soups and shakes, but this could end up having too much sugar for bypass patients

- Rice Dream milk

- Oatly, or oat-based drinks

- V8 or tomato juice

- Diluted fruit juice

- Mashed potatoes that are mixed with gravy or broth with the consistency of soup

- Whey protein isolate powder combined with milk or water and frozen into ice cream

- Whey protein isolate drinks

- Smooth cream-style soups, low in fat

- Unsweetened plain yogurt without sugar or fruit added

- Milky chai type tea

- Milk – almond, soy, semi-skim, or skim

Recipes

Mocha Frappuccino

Ingredients

Low-sugar chocolate syrup – optional

Low-fat whipped cream – optional

1 c ice

1 tbsp. cocoa powder

3 to 4 drops liquid sweetener

½ c 0% fat Greek yogurt

¼ c unsweetened almond milk

¼ c brewed coffee

Directions

Put the ice, cocoa, sweetener, yogurt, milk, and coffee into your blender and whizz everything together until it is smooth.

Pour the mixture into a mug or glass and swirl in the chocolate syrup and whipped cream. Enjoy.

Coco-Rita Cocktail

Ingredients

2 tbsps. orange juice, fresh

4 tbsps. coconut water

2 tbsps. birch syrup – or favorite sugar-free syrup

5 tbsps. lime juice, fresh

Rock salt – garnish

Lime wedge

Directions

Pick your favorite martini glass, run the lime wedge around the rim and dip it into the rock salt.

Shake the orange juice, coconut water, syrup, and lime juice vigorously together.

Strain the drink into your glass and enjoy.

5-A-Day Smoothie

Ingredients

2/3 c orange juice, fresh

¼ avocado, chopped and peeled

5 tbsps. low-fat coconut milk

Handful spinach leaves

1 dessert pear

1 apple

Directions

Remove the cores from the pear and apple, and slice them into small pieces.

In your blender, add the orange juice, avocado, coconut milk, spinach, pear, and apple. Pulse the mixture together until it is well blended.

Pour the mixture into a glass and enjoy.

Curry Root Soup

Ingredients

Mint leaves, Greek yogurt, and mango chutney for garnish – optional

Squeeze lemon juice

5 c vegetable stock

1 to 2 tsp curry powder

Pepper

2 crushed garlic cloves

Salt

1 lb. carrots, chopped and peeled

1 lb. rutabaga and swede, chopped and peeled

2 leeks, sliced

1 onion, chopped and peeled

Low-fat cooking spray or a little oil

Directions

Place the cooking spray or oil in your skillet and let it warm up. Place the carrots, rutabaga or swede, leeks, and onion in the skillet and sprinkle with the pepper and salt. Let this gently cook for 30 minutes. Give it a stir now and then. Add a touch of water or oil if it looks like it becomes dry. You want the veggies to soften, but their colors should change too much.

Mix in the curry powder and garlic and let this mixture cook for a couple of minutes.

Pour in the stock and allow the mixture to boil. Turn the heat down and let the mixture simmer for about 15 minutes.

In small batches, place the soup in your blender and mix until it is completely thick and smooth. You can use an immersion blender if available. Blend everything in the pot and mix until smooth.

Place everything back in the pan, add the lemon juice. Taste and adjust the flavorings as you need. Serve in a mug or a bowl.

Pumpkin Pie Shake

Ingredients

½ c ice

1 tbsp. pecans

½ tsp cinnamon

1 c nut milk

1 scoop pumpkin pie protein milkshake

Directions

Using a blender, mix all of the ingredients listed above. Blend until you get a smooth consistency. Then, pour the mixture into a glass and enjoy.

Oatmeal Cookie Shake

Ingredients

Squirt low-fat cream, nuts, and cinnamon for garnish – optional

Ice – optional

¼ tsp vanilla

1 scoop vanilla whey protein powder

1 tbsp. oatmeal

½ tsp cinnamon

1 c low-fat nut milk

Directions

Put the ice, vanilla, oatmeal, cinnamon, milk, and protein powder into your blender and pulse a few times until smooth.

Place the mixture into a glass and serve with some nuts, cinnamon, and low-fat cream.

Apple Strudel Shake

Ingredients

Drizzle of sugar-free syrup and squirt of low-fat cream – option

1 scoop vanilla whey protein powder

1 tsp raisins – optional

¼ tsp cinnamon

3 tbsps. unsweetened applesauce

1 c low-fat nut milk

Directions

Put the cinnamon, applesauce, milk, protein powder, and the raisins if you want to use them, into your blender and pulse a few times until mixed.

Place the mixture into a glass and top with sugar-free syrup and low-fat cream, and enjoy.

Berkshire Iced Tea

Ingredients

Mint sprig and lemon slice for garnish

Ice

1 tbsp. rum – optional

1 tbsp. vodka – optional

¼ c 100% grapefruit juice

1 c boiling water

Ginger and lemon flavored tea bag

Directions

Put the tea bag into the water and let the mixture steep for at least five minutes. Take the tea bag out of the water and discard in. Let the mixture cool.

Once everything is cool, add in the grapefruits juice, if you are still in the first stages after surgery, or you can add in the run and vodka if you have been cleared to drink alcohol.

Place into a glass full of ice and garnish with mint sprig and lemon slice.

Cinnamon Spice Shake

Ingredients

1 scoop protein powder – cinnamon bun flavored, or vanilla with a teaspoon of cinnamon

¼ c applesauce, unsweetened

1 c unsweetened almond milk or low-fat skim milk

Directions

Place the protein powder, with or without the cinnamon, applesauce, and milk into your blender and pulse a few times until mixed.

Pour the mixture into a glass and top with a dusting of cinnamon.

Banana Bomb

Ingredients

½ banana, frozen

2 scoops vanilla protein powder

4 oz. almond milk, unsweetened

4 oz. Greek yogurt, fat-free

Directions

Blend all the ingredients using a blender. Blend until you get a smooth consistency.

Dispense the mixture into your favorite glass and top with some pistachios and banana slices if desired.

Fro-Yo Popsicles

Ingredients

2 c strawberries, hulled

2 c Greek yogurt, full-fat – use fat-free if you want or need to, but the full-fat makes for a firmer texture

Directions

Put both of the above ingredients into your blender and puree them together until they are completely smooth.

Spoon this mixture into popsicle molds, or plastic cups with sticks, and place them in the freeze for at least four to six hours, or overnight for the best results

Unmold the popsicles and enjoy.

Frappuccino with Protein

Ingredients

No-cal sweetener – optional

1 ½ c crushed ice

¼ tsp cinnamon

1 scoop vanilla protein powder

½ c vanilla almond milk, unsweetened

3 tbsps. hot water

1 ½ tsp coffee granules, instant

Directions

Stir the water and the coffee granules together until they are fully dissolved. Place the sweetener, ice, cinnamon, protein powder, milk, and coffee into your blender.

Set the blender to ice speed and mix until smooth. You may end up having to press puree a few times, or stir it depending on how your blender works. As you blend the mixture it will become frothier, so mix until it gets to the consistency that you like.

Place the mixture into a glass, top with some nonfat cream if you want, and enjoy.

Jello Cups

Ingredients

Mint sprig and low-fat whipped cream for garnish – optional

1 c fat-free Greek yogurt

1 ¼ c raspberries

1 oz. packet sugar-free jello crystals

Directions

Mix the jello crystals into 3 ¾ cups of boiling water and mix until they have dissolved. Let the mixture cool, but make sure it doesn't set.

Once it is cold, mix in the yogurt and beat until it is combined.

Spread the raspberries into four serving cups. Place the prepared jello over the berries and place in the refrigerator until it has set up.

Serve with a mint sprig and whipped cream if you want.

Egg Nog

Ingredients

2 bananas

Couple drops rum extract

3 eggs, separated

1 tsp nutmeg

Vanilla pod

2 cinnamon sticks

1 ¾ c milk, skim

Directions

Put the nutmeg, seeds from the vanilla pot, cinnamon stick, and milk in a pot. Let the mixture come up to a boil. Let the mixture cool and completely chill. Once it is chilled strain the milk mixture.

Put the yolks into a blender, rum extract, and bananas. Puree the mixture together until smooth. Pour the milk mixture into the blender and combine. It's ready to enjoy, or you can place it in the fridge until you need it, up to 48 hours.

Once ready to drink, whisk up the egg whites until they form stiff peaks. Mix this into the milk mixture. Place into a glass and top with a dusting of nutmeg if you want.

California Prune

Ingredients

1 tbsps. no-sugar added peanut butter

1 tsp wheat germ

1 c berry fruits – canned, fresh, or frozen

2/3 c milk, skim

2/3 California prune juice

1 banana

Directions

Place all of the above ingredients into your blender and mix until it becomes smooth.

Pour half of the smoothie into a serving glass and place the rest in the fridge to have later.

Pumpkin Soup

Ingredients

Pepper

Salt

1 ¾ c vegetable bouillon or stock

2 pcs of ginger, grated

14 oz. coconut milk, reduced fat

1 ½ lb. squash or pumpkin flesh, cubed

2 tsp curry powder

3 crushed garlic cloves

1 large onion or 3 shallots, chopped

Low-fat cooking spray

Directions

Use a generous amount of the low-fat spray to coat a large pan. Let the pan heat up and add the onion or shallot and let it cook for three to four minutes until it has softened up.

Mix in the curry powder, garlic, and ginger and let this cook for another minute. Next, mix in the squash or pumpkin flesh, stock, and coconut milk. Let the mixture come up to a boil, turn down the heat, and then let it simmer for 10 to 12 minutes. The squash or pumpkin should be tender.

Using an immersion blender, blend up the soup mixture until it is completely smooth. You can use a blender or food processor if immersion blender is unavailable. Add salt and pepper according to your taste, and place back on the heat until hot. Serve with a sprinkling of toasted pumpkin seeds if you can tolerate them.

Carrot and Sweet Potato Soup

Ingredients

Grated carrot, snipped chives, and fat-free yogurt for garnish – optional

Pepper

Salt

6 c vegetable stock

1 tsp cumin

1 in piece ginger, grated

1 lb. carrots, chopped and peeled

2 lb. sweet potato, chopped and peeled

Low-fat cooking spray

Directions

Place a generous amount of the nonstick spray on your pan and let the pan heat up. Add the cumin, ginger, carrots, and sweet potato and let it cook for about ten minutes. Make sure you occasionally stir so that everything begins to brown.

Pour in the stock and then add the pepper and salt according to your taste, let the mixture come to a boil. Place on the lid and let the mixture simmer for around 40 minutes, or until the vegetables turn tender.

Using an immersion blender, blend up the soup mixture until it is completely smooth. If you don't have one, you can add batches of the soup into a regular blender or food processor until smooth. Place back into the pan and let everything heat back up.

Serve the soup with a sprinkle of herbs and some plain yogurt if you would like.

Pumpkin Spice Smoothie

Ingredients

Squirt sugar-free whipped cream – optional

2 scoops espresso protein drink

1 c cold water

¼ tsp vanilla

½ tsp pumpkin pie spice

½ c low-fat milk

Directions

Put the vanilla, pumpkin pie spice, and milk in a shaker. Seal the lid and shake it until it is blended.

Pour in the espresso protein drink and the water. Seal the lid and shake it again until well mixed.

Place the mixture into a serving glass and top with some sugar-free whipped cream if you would like.

Ham and Pea Soup

Ingredients

Mint and pea shoots for garnish

Pepper

Salt

2 oz. fresh pea shoots

2 tbsps. chopped mint

¼ c cooked bacon or ham, chopped

4 oz. frozen peas

1 stick celery, chopped

3 ¾ c hot vegetable stock or bouillon

5 to 6 new potatoes, with skins and chopped

2 tbsps. light butter

1 onion, chopped

Directions

Place the butter in a pot and allow it to melt. Mix in the potatoes, celery, and onion and allow this cook for about five more minutes.

Pour in the bouillon or stock and allow it to simmer for another 15 minutes or until the potatoes are fork tender.

Mix in the peas and return it to a simmer and cook for another five minutes.

Remove the pot from the heat and mix in the mint and pea shoots, and then the bacon or ham. Stir everything together.

Mix the soup using an immersion blender. Blend until you get a smooth consistency. As an alternative, you can use a blender or food processor and blend the soup by batch. Dash some pepper and salt according to your taste.

Place back in the pot and let the soup heat back up. Garnish with mint and pea shoots if you would like.

Spiced Carrot and Parsnip Soup

Ingredients

1 tsp cumin seeds, toasted – optional

Pepper

Salt

1 orange, zest, and juice

4 ¼ c hot vegetable bouillon or stock

1 lb. carrots, cubed and peeled

1 tbsp. garam masala

1 to 2 red chilies, chopped and deseeded

1 onion, chopped

Low-fat cooking spray

Directions

Spray a large pot with a generous amount of the nonstick spray. Let the pot heat up and then mix in the chili and onion and allow it to cook for five minutes until they are soft. Mix in the garam masala and let it all cook for another minute.

Mix in a cup of water, stock, carrots, and parsnips. Let the mixture come to boil and place on the lid. Let the mixture simmer for 20 to 25 minutes, or until the veggies have become tender.

Using an immersion blender, mix up the soup until it is smooth. As an alternative, you can use a food processor or blender. Add the pepper, orange juice, salt, and orange zest. Place back in the pot over the heat and let it warm back up. Serve with cumin seeds if you would like.

Shamrock Smoothie

Ingredients

Mint sprigs, garnish

1 oz. unflavored protein powder – optional

2 tbsps. lime juice, fresh

1 kiwi fruit, sliced and peeled

2 c cantaloupe, cubed and frozen

Directions

Put the protein powder, if you using, lime juice, kiwi, and melon in your blender and mix in up until everything has blended

Split the smoothie between two glasses. Top with some mint sprigs and enjoy.

Carrot, Lentil, and Apple Soup

Ingredients

4 tbsps. cilantro, chopped, for garnish

4 tbsps. Greek yogurt, fat-free, for garnish

Pepper

Salt

1 c coconut milk, light

3 c hot vegetable bouillon

2/3 c split red lentils

1 celery stalk, sliced finely

2 apples, cored, peeled, and chopped

1 lb. carrots, cut and peeled

Low-fat cooking spray

2 tsp cumin seeds

½ tsp chili flakes

Directions

Get a large pot heated and add in the cumin seeds and the chili flakes. Let this dry-fry for a minute, or until you start to smell their aroma and they start to pop. Take out half of the seeds, leaving the rest in the pot.

Add a generous amount of the nonstick spray, and let it heat. Add in the celery, apple, and carrots. Let this mixture cook for around five minutes and then mix in the coconut milk, bouillon or stock, and lentils. Let the mixture come up to a simmer, place on the lid, and let it cook for about 15 minutes. The lentils and carrots should be tender.

Use an immersion blender to puree the mixture until smooth. If you don't have one, place small amounts in a regular blender and mixture it up until all is smooth. Add in pepper and salt to your taste.

Serve the soup with cilantro and some yogurt. Add on some of the reserved spices.

Pumpkin Pepper Soup

Ingredients

1 tbsp. toasted pumpkin seeds

2 tsp fresh chives, chopped

4 tbsps. Greek yogurt, fat-free

Pepper

Salt

5 c strong vegetable stock

1 tsp thyme leaves

4 garlic cloves, crushed and peeled

1 red chili, chopped and deseeded

1 ½ lb. pumpkin, diced and peeled

6 shallots, chopped and peeled

Low-fat cooking spray

4 red peppers, quartered and deseeded

Directions

Your oven should be set to 400.

Put the red peppers, with skin side up, onto a baking sheet and place them in the oven to roast for 20 to 25 minutes, or until the skin has charred up. Take them off the baking sheet and put them in a bowl. Cover the bowl with saran wrap and let the peppers cool. After they are cooled, peel the skins off and keep the fresh flesh.

While the peppers are getting ready, spray your skillet with a cooking spray. As an alternative, you can brush the skillet with butter or cooking oil. Let the skillet heat up and add in the red chili, pumpkin, and shallots. Let them cook for five to ten minutes, or until everything has softened up.

Mix in the thyme and garlic and let it cook for another minute. Pour in the stock and allow the mixture to boil. Turn the heat down and place on the lid, allowing it to simmer for about 15 minutes.

Place the pepper, red peppers, and salt and let it cook for another five minutes.

Finish up the soup by blending it with an immersion blender or a regular blender until completely smooth. Taste the soup and adjust any of the flavorings that you need to. Place the soup back over the heat, and heat it back to hot. Serve the soup with some pumpkin seeds, chives, and yogurt.

Cauliflower Cheese Soup

Ingredients

Grated nutmegs, pepper, and salt for seasoning

1 ½ c grated hard cheese, low-fat

3 ¾ c milk, skim

2 garlic cloves, chopped

1 potato, large

1 head cauliflower, small to medium

Directions

Trim up, wash, and then chop up the cauliflower, getting rid of the rough stalks. Peel the potato and then finely chop.

Put the milk, garlic, potato, and cauliflower in the skillet and let it heat up on low. Let the mixture simmer until the potato pieces have become fork tender. This will take around ten to 12 minutes.

Mix in the nutmegs, pepper, cheese, and salt and use an immersion blender to mix up the soup until smooth. You can also place it in a regular blender and mix until smooth. Make sure it's piping hot before you serve, or serve at room temperature.

Pink Lady Lollies

Ingredients

6 tbsps. Splenda

1 lb. frozen or fresh mixed summer or forest berry fruits

2 apples, pink lady

Directions

Core, peel, and chop up the apples and place them in a pan with four tablespoons of water. Let them cook for about four minutes.

Add in the berries and let it cook for another three minutes.

Take them off the heat and then mix in the sweetener until it has dissolved. Taste the mixture and add more sweetener if you need to.

Mix this up in a blender and strain to get rid of the seeds. Let the mixture cool and place them in popsicle molds. Allow them to freeze overnight until they have firmed up.

Pea and Leek Soup

Ingredients

Leek twists and mint sprigs for garnish – optional

½ lb. soft cheese, fat-free

Pepper

Salt

½ lb. peas, frozen

4 ¼ c vegetable stock or bouillon

1 tsp olive oil

1 tbsp. low-fat spread

20 mint leaves, chopped

2 lettuce hearts, chopped

1 ¼ lb. medium leeks, chopped and trimmed

Directions

Place the oil, spread, mint, lettuce, and leeks in a large skillet. Let this gently warm up until everything starts to soften.

Mix in the bouillon or stock and let it simmer for five minutes. Mix in the pepper, peas, and salt. Let this cook for another five minutes.

Pour this mixture into a blender along with the cheese and mix until smooth. Place back into the skillet and let everything warm together. Do not let this mixture come to a boil.

Serve cold or warm with a garnish of leeks and mint.

Red Thai Pumpkin Soup

Ingredients

Chopped cilantro for garnish – optional

Lime juice

Pepper

Salt

3 tbsps. red Thai curry paste

2 ½ c vegetable stock

1 can pumpkin

1 ¾ c coconut milk, reduced fat

1 tsp chopped lemongrass – optional

1 tbsp. ginger, chopped

1 onion, chopped and peeled

Light cooking spray

Directions

Coat a large skillet with some cooking spray. Mix in the lemongrass, if using, ginger, and onion and let it cook for at least ten minutes, or until everything has softened.

Mix in the pepper, curry paste, salt, stock, pumpkin, and coconut milk, and combine well. Place on the lid and allow the mixture to cook for 15 minutes. Occasionally stir the mixture.

Pour everything into your blender and mix it up until smooth. Place back in the skillet and let everything heat through. Add a little squeeze of lime to the dish and top with some chopped cilantro.

Cheesy Broccoli Soup

Ingredients

Croutons – optional
Pepper
Salt
5.2 oz. dolcelatte cheese
4 1/3 vegetable stock
2 7 oz. packs of broccoli
Bay leaf
1 potato, diced and peeled
2 garlic cloves, crushed
1 onion, chopped
Light cooking spray

Directions

Generously spray a skillet with cooking spray. Place in the onion and cook for five minutes until it has softened, but the color should not change. Stir in the bay leaf, garlic, and potato. Place on the lid and let it cook for another five minutes. Stir occasionally until the potatoes have softened.

While that's cooking, chop the broccoli up into small pieces and place them in the skillet along with the stock. Let everything come up to a simmer and continue to cook for around five minutes or until the broccoli becomes tender. Chop up the dolcelatte roughly and mix it into the skillet until it is soft.

Take out the bay leaf. With either a regular blender or an immersion blender, mix up the soup until smooth. Add in pepper and salt to your tasting.

Serve with croutons if you would like.

Turkish Mint Soup

Ingredients

Pepper

Salt

2 1/5 c vegetable stock

Handful mint, chopped

14 oz. lentils

14 oz. tomatoes, chopped

1 garlic clove, crushed

1 onion, chopped

Light cooking spray

Directions

Coat a pan with some of the cooking spray. Place the garlic and onion and let them cook until they have softened around three to five minutes.

Mix in the pepper, stock, salt, entire contents of lentils can, and tomatoes.

Let the mixture boil. Reduce the heat and cover with lid. Let it simmer for another 15 to 20 minutes.

Place the mixture into your blender and mix until it is completely smooth.

Beetroot Smoothie

Ingredients

1 beetroot, cooked

½ c orange juice

½ c pomegranate juice

Directions

Place all of the above ingredients into your blender and whizz it all together.

Strawberry Kiwi Smoothie

Ingredients

½ c low-fat milk

1 banana, sliced

1 kiwi fruit, chopped and peeled

3 strawberries, large

Directions

Process the banana, strawberries, milk, and kiwi together in your blender until it is smooth.

Egg Custard

Ingredients

½ tsp vanilla

4 tbsps. Splenda

4 egg yolks

2 ½ c milk, skim

Directions

Place the milk in a heavy pot and let it come up to a boil.

Using a large bowl, beat the Splenda and yolks together until they are creamy.

Place the milk into the whipped yolks, and beat together until well blended. Rinse out the pot.

Strain the egg mixture through a sieve and put it back into the pot and cook at a low temp. Let it cook while you constantly stir until everything has started to thicken up to where it will coat your spoon and has a heavy cream consistency.

Serve as it is, cold, or with a dusting of nutmeg. You can also add bananas or fruit puree if you are in the stage to handle them.

Chocolate Ice Cream

Ingredients

2 tbsps. hot chocolate powder, low-fat

2/3 c milk, skim

2/3 c custard, low-fat

2 scoops flavorless protein powder

4-4 oz. vanilla and chocolate yogurt

Directions

Combine the chocolate powder, milk, custard, protein powder, and the yogurt.

Place the mixture in the freezer and freeze until it has firmed up. Make sure you check every so often and whisk it up a few times before it is completely hard. This makes sure that it doesn't form large ice crystals. You can use an ice cream maker to freeze it if available.

Let it soften for about 30 minutes before serving.

Mango Smoothie

Ingredients

2/3 c milk, reduced-fat or skim

1 scoop protein powder

½ mango, chopped and peeled

Directions

Place all of the above ingredients in your blender and mix until it is completely smooth.

Banana and Coconut Puree

Ingredients

¼ tsp cinnamon

1 to 2 tbsps. canned coconut milk, low-fat

½ banana, peeled

Directions

Put the bananas in a bowl and mash them up with a fork until it is about smooth.

Place the banana in the microwave and set it for 10 seconds, stir it around, and heat it for another 10 seconds. Continue this until it is warmed through.

Mix in the cinnamon and coconut milk.

This can store in the fridge for one day, or you can freeze it up for three months.

Cheeseburger Soup

Ingredients

16 oz. Velveeta cheese, cubed, or 2 c shredded cheddar

½ tsp pepper

½ tsp salt

2 c milk, skim

¼ c AP flour

3 tbsps. butter

1 lb. ground beef, lean

3 c chicken broth

1 tsp parsley, dried

1 tsp basil, dried

½ c celery, diced

1 c carrots, shredded

1 small onion, chopped

4 small potatoes, diced and peeled

Directions

Put the parsley, basil, celery, carrots, onions, and potatoes in your slow cooker. Add in the broth. Place on the slow cooker lid. Set your cooker to a low heat and set it for six to eight hour, or, if you need it done faster, you can set your cooker to high for four to five hours. The potatoes should be tender.

At around 45 minutes before you plan on enjoying your soup, you should cook the beef and place it into your cooker. Wipe out the skillet you used and melt the butter. Whisk the flour into the butter and let it cook until it becomes browned and bubbly. Stir in your milk, pepper, and salt. Place this into your slow cooker and stir everything together.

Add the cheese, Velveeta or shredded, and stir everything together well. Place the lid on the cooker and let it cook for another 30 minutes. You can enjoy it like this if you can eat solid foods. If you are still in the liquid/pureed phase, take your immersion blender and blend it up until it is smooth.

Buffalo Chicken Dip

Ingredients

1 c mozzarella, reduced-fat

2 c shredded chicken, cooked

2/3 c hot sauce

2 tbsps. ranch dip seasoning – optional spicy flavor

1 c 0% Greek yogurt

10 oz. Neufchatel cream cheese, room temp

Directions

You should place all of the above ingredients into your slow cooker. It is best to use a slow cooker liner in this process as t can make everything a lot easier.

You should set the cooker to low at three to four hours. Make sure you stir it every hour.

Once this is done, make sure that the chicken is shredded and mashed up enough, and that there is enough liquid so that it has a thin consistency.

Cauliflower Cheese Soup

Ingredients

Cilantro – optional

1/8 tsp cayenne

Pepper

Salt

5 ½ oz. sharp white cheddar, grated

4 c chicken broth, plus a little extra if needed

1 head cauliflower, medium, trimmed and cut into small pieces

1 large onion, diced

3 tbsps. butter

Directions

Place the butter into a big pot and let it melt. Mix in the onion and let it cook until it has softened; make sure that you stir often. Place in the cauliflower and let it cook until it starts to brown up. This will likely take about 12 minutes.

Add in a cup of water and the broth and let the mixture come to a boil. Lower the amount of heat and let the mixture continue to cook until the cauliflower until it is tender. This will take around 20 minutes. Let this mixture cool and little.

Place batches of the mixture into a blender and mix it until smooth. Continue doing this until you puree all of the soup. Make sure you are careful because the soup will still be hot.

Place everything back into your big pot, and add in some more water or broth to thin it out a bit if you need to.

Let everything heat through and mix in the cheese, stirring until it has melted completely. Add the pepper, salt, and a little sprinkle of cayenne.

Garnish the soup with cilantro if you would like.

Pureed Pintos

Ingredients

½ c chicken broth

2 cloves garlic, chopped

1 c salsa

1 medium onion, diced

15 oz. pinto beans, rinsed and drained

2 tsp olive oil

Directions

Cook your garlic and onion in a skillet until they have browned up slightly. Place the beans, salsa, and the cooked veggies into your blender. You can also use a food processor if you have. Slowly add in a little chicken broth until it becomes smooth enough for you to eat. Place the mixture into the pan and let it cook until it begins to bubble and bit and heats through.

Soft Eggs with Chives and Ricotta

Ingredients

Olive oil

1 tbsp. chives, chopped

½ c ricotta

½ c milk

2 eggs

Directions

Place the milk and the eggs into a jar. Top with its lid and shake with all your might to scramble the mixture together.

Warm up your skillet and place in the scrambled eggs. Cook and stir the eggs until they become soft-set. Stir the eggs gently now and then.

Once they are just set, mix in the chives and the ricotta. Place the eggs on a plate and serve with a little drizzle of oil if you would like.

Mashed Cauliflower

Ingredients

Pepper

Salt

¼ c chives, chopped

¼ c parmesan, grated

2 c chicken broth

2 small cauliflower heads, cored and cut into florets

Directions

Place the broth and the cauliflower into a pot and let the mixture start to boil. Lower the pots temp and place on the lid. Allow this mixture to continue to cook for around 15 to 20 minutes. The cauliflower needs to be tender, but it should be falling apart.

With a slotted spoon, place the cauliflower into your food processor and mix it until it is completely smooth. Place this into a bowl and mix in the chives and parmesan. Add the pepper and the salt, and mix until it is smooth.

Ricotta Bake

Ingredients

½ c mozzarella, shredded, part skim

½ c marinara sauce

Pepper

Salt

1 tsp Italian seasoning

1 egg, beaten

½ parmesan, grated

8 oz. ricotta cheese, part skim

Directions

Place the seasonings, egg, parmesan, and the ricotta in a bowl and mix it together very well. Pour the mixture into a baking dish that has been coated with cooking spray. Place the marinara sauce over the top and add on the mozzarella cheese. Your oven should be set at 450 and place in the baking dish and let the mixture cook for 20 to 25 minutes. It should become brown and bubbly.

Deviled Egg Salad

Ingredients

Toasted bread – optional

Lettuce – optional

Pepper

Salt

1 tsp garlic powder

1 tsp onion powder

1 tbsp. pickle relish

1 tsp mustard

½ c miracle whip

6 eggs

Directions

Place the six eggs in a pot and fill it up with water. Let the water start to boil and time them to cook for 15 minutes. Once they are done, drain the water, crack the eggs slightly, and let them sit in cold water until cool enough for you to touch.

Peel the cooked eggs and dice them up into smaller bits. Mix the in the miracle whip and all of the other spices until well mixed.

If you want, place this on a slice of toast or lettuce.

Salmon Pate

Ingredients

1/8 tsp pepper

1/8 tsp salt

1 tbsp. lemon juice

½ tsp dill, dried

2 tbsps. 0% fat Greek yogurt

2.5 oz. smoked salmon

Directions

Place the above ingredients, except for the yogurt, into your food processor. Mix everything up until the fish has been diced up finely.

Place the diced fish in a bowl and stir in the yogurt until everything is smooth.

Southwest Bean Dip

Ingredients

1 c pinto beans, drained

1/3 c salsa

¼ c cilantro

½ c Mexican cheese blend

Directions

Place the beans, salsa, and the cilantro in your food processor until it only has a little bit of texture. Pour this mixture into your baking dish and top, or stir the cheese into the bean mixture. Your oven should be set at 350. Let the mixture cook for 25 to 30 minutes.

Cheesecake Protein Pudding

Ingredients

1 pkg cheesecake pudding mix, sugar-free

1 scoop vanilla protein powder – Bari-essentials or Bari-Clear

1 c Greek yogurt

Directions

Place all of the above ingredients into your blender and mix together until completely smooth.

Lemon Ricotta Creme

Ingredients

4 packets Splenda

1 ½ tsp vanilla

1 to 2 tsp lemon extract – or orange

1 lemon, zest – or orange

15 oz. ricotta cheese, low-fat or fat-free

Directions

Place everything from the above list into your blender and whirr until they are all smooth and combined.

Refried Bean Soup

Ingredients

16 oz. refried beans

8 oz. ground beef, browned and mixed with ½ packet taco seasoning

1 small onion

1 medium tomato

4 tbsps. green chili peppers

11 oz. Mexican style corn

½ packet taco seasoning

2 c chicken broth

Directions

Place the tomato, onion, beef, and refried beans in your food processor and pulse until they become slightly chopped.

Place this mixture into a pot and add the broth, taco seasoning, and corn and stir together. Let this mixture come up to a boil and cook for about 15 minutes.

Pepperoni Pizza Casserole

Ingredients

½ c mozzarella, shredded

12 pepperoni slices

Pepper

Salt

¼ c mozzarella, shredded

8 pepperoni slices

1 tbsp. butter

2 tbsps. heavy cream

1 head cauliflower

Directions

Clean up the cauliflower and break it into small pieces. Put this in a bowl with the butter and cream. Place this in the microwave, keeping it uncovered, and microwave for ten minutes. Stir the cauliflower so that it gets coated with the cream and butter. Microwave for another six minutes, or until the cauliflower has become tender. Take the tender cauliflower and place it into your food processor as well as a quarter cup of mozzarella, and eight pepperoni slices. Pulse the mixture until it is smooth. Add in pepper and salt according to your taste. You can also adjust the cream and butter to suit your preferences.

Place the mixture into an eight by eight baking dish. Add in a half cup mozzarella and top with the pepperoni. Your oven should be set at 375. Bake the mixture for 20 minutes.

Avocado Potato Puree

Ingredients

Pepper

Salt

2 tsp milk, skim

½ avocado, peeled

2 oz. chicken breast or thigh, boneless and skinless

1 small potato, peeled and chunked

Directions

Cook the chicken and the potato together until the both are cooked through, and the potato is fork tender.

Put this in a blender along with the pepper, salt, milk, and avocado. Mix this up until it smooth. If you need it to be thinner, add in some milk. Adjust the flavors to your taste.

Diner Chicken Salad

Ingredients

¼ tsp pepper

½ tsp salt

2 celery stalks, diced finely

1 tsp mustard

¾ c mayonnaise, light olive oil

2 12oz cans chicken, shredded finely

¼ onion, diced finely

Directions

Put all of this into a bowl and stir it together. Season as you need and adjust the amount of mayo to how creamy you want your chicken salad.

Crab Spread

Ingredients

1 can crab meat, shredded

1 tsp garlic powder

¼ tsp horseradish

1 tbsp. hot mustard

¼ c cheddar cheese, shredded

1 tbsp. Bari-Clear protein powder

¼ c light mayonnaise

½ c cottage cheese, fat-free

¼ c cream cheese, fat-free

Directions

Put the crab meat, cottage cheese, and cream cheese into your food processor and mix it up until it is smooth. Place in a bowl and then stir in all of the remaining ingredients. Place in the microwave for three to five minutes. Allow this to cool for five minutes before you eat it.

Cheese Lasagna

Ingredients

¼ c mozzarella, 2% milk

2 egg whites

¼ tsp basil

¼ tsp oregano

¼ c marinara

¾ c cottage cheese, fat-free

Directions

Combine the basil, oregano, egg whites, and cottage cheese together and put this all in a baking dish. Pour the marinara sauce all over the mixture and then sprinkle on the mozzarella. Your oven should be at 450, and you should cook it for 20 minutes.

Squash Casserole

Ingredients

1 scoop Bari-Clear protein powder

1 tbsp. cheddar cheese, shredded

1 to 2 tsp butter

Pepper

Salt

½ tsp garlic powder

2 tbsps. cream cheese, fat-free

1 can squash with Vidalia

Directions

Put all of the above ingredients into your blender and mix until it is smooth. Pour the mixture into a bowl and let it microwave for 90 seconds.

Parmesan Cauliflower

Ingredients

1 tbsp. bari-clear protein powder

¼ c milk

¼ c parmesan

¼ c mozzarella

¼ tsp pepper

¼ tsp garlic powder

1 tsp salt

1 bag cauliflower florets

Directions

Put the bari-clear, milk, parmesan, pepper, salt, garlic, and cauliflower in your blender and mix until it has become smooth. Place this into a large bowl and add on some mozzarella cheese, and place it in the microwave for 90 seconds.

Enchilada Eggs

Ingredients

Pinch salt

4 eggs

10 oz. enchilada sauce

½ can refried black beans, fat-free

Directions

Place the refried black beans into a pot and let the heat up to a simmer.

In a different skillet, place in the enchilada sauce and let it heat up.

Make four different wells in the enchilada sauce. Gently crack one of the eggs into each of the wells that you just made. Place a covering on the skillet and let the eggs cook for about five minutes if you like soft yolks or if you want them firm.

Place some of the refried beans on a plate and then top with sauce and egg.

Italian Poached Eggs

Ingredients

4 basil leaves, shredded

Pepper

Salt

4 eggs

3 to 4 pieces roasted red pepper, sliced

16 oz. marinara sauce

Directions

Heat up a large skillet and place in the peppers and the marinara sauce.

With a spoon, make a well into the sauce mixture, and repeat this process three more times. Take your eggs, and crack one of them into each of the wells.

Top the eggs with some pepper and salt.

Let this mixture cook for around 12 minutes, or until the eggs have cooked to your desired firmness. You can also cover them if you wish for them to cook slightly faster.

Take the skillet off of the heats and add the torn basil. Scoop out an egg with some sauce and enjoy.

Creamy Deviled Eggs

Ingredients

Dash paprika

Dash pepper

¼ tsp salt

Splash pickle juice

2 tsp mustard

½ c mayonnaise, low-fat

8 eggs

Directions

Place the eggs into a pot and fill it up with water so that the eggs are covered. Set this over heat and allow the water to come up to a boil. Once they are boiling, cook them for 15 minutes. After their done, drain off the water and slightly crack the eggs and cover in cold water.

Once the eggs have cooled to a temp that you can handle, peel them, and slice them in half lengthwise. Carefully take the eggs out and place them in a bowl. Mash up the yolks and stir in the seasonings, mustard, pickle juice, and mayonnaise.

You can use a piping bag for this part if you want otherwise use a spoon to disperse this mixture between the 16 egg halves evenly. Sprinkle the tops with some paprika.

Deviled Egg Dip

Ingredients

3 green onions, sliced and divided

1 tbsp. Dijon mustard

1 tbsp. white vinegar

4 triangles creamy Swiss, Laughing Cow Cheese

½ c mayonnaise, fat-free

8 eggs, hard boiled, divided

Directions

Set one of your cooked eggs aside for use later. Slice all of the eggs along the long side, just like if you were going to make deviled eggs, and take out the yolks, placing them in a food processor. Place in the mustard, vinegar, cheese wedges, mayonnaise, and half of the white parts of the eggs. Mix until the mixture until it is smooth. Scoop this out into a serving bowl.

Chop the rest of the egg whites up and then mix it into the dip as well as 2/3 of the onions.

Take the egg you reserved earlier and chop it up. Add this across the top of the dip with the rest of the green onions. Once you are on regular food, you can serve this with veggies.

Creamy Vegetable Soup

Ingredients

¼ c half and half or coconut milk

3 sprigs thyme – or 1 tsp dried thyme

2 bay leaves

3 c chicken stock

1 tbsp. olive oil

3 cloves garlic, halved and peeled

1 lb. thin skin potatoes

¼ tsp crushed red pepper flakes

Salt

4 celery sticks

1 lb. carrots, peeled

1 large onion

Directions

Chop up the celery, potatoes onion, and carrots into half inch chunks. Set the potatoes to the side by their self away from the other vegetables.

Place oil into a big pot and let it heat up until it shimmers. Add in the celery, onion, and carrots and mix them around in the oil. Add a half teaspoon of salt and the pepper flakes. Let this cook until the vegetables start to sweat, soften up, and the begin smelling sweet. This will take around five to ten minutes.

Mix in the thyme, bay leaves, garlic, and potatoes. Let this mixture cook for another five minutes. If your pot seems dry add in a little bit of oil.

Pour the stock over everything and allow the mixture come up to a boil. Let the heat turn down to a simmer and let it continue to cook until you can easily break into a potato with a fork. This will take about 15 minutes.

To finish up the soup, take it off of the heat. Remove the sprigs of thyme and the bay leaves. If you have an immersion blender, use it up to smooth out the soup, if not, places batches into a regular blender until all of the soup has become smooth.

Mix in the half and half or coconut milk. Taste the soup and adjust any of the flavorings that you need.

Pineapple Dip

Ingredients

1 c plain yogurt, fat-free

4 c pineapple, frozen

Directions

Place both of the above ingredients into your food processor; you can use a blender if you don't have a food processor.

Pulse up the mixture until it is completely smooth and creamy.

Enjoy.

Pumpkin Cheesecake Pudding

Ingredients

2 tsp pumpkin pie spice

2 scoops vanilla protein powder

1 ½ c milk, skim

2 packs cheesecake pudding mix, sugar-free

1 container cool whip, sugar-free

1 can pumpkin puree – do not get pumpkin pie filling

Directions

Place all of the above ingredients into a bowl. Use a hand mixer and beat it all together until it is all smooth.

Allow the mixture to sit in the fridge for a little while.

Cauliflower Casserole

Ingredients

¼ c bread crumbs – optional

¾ lb. sharp cheddar cheese

3 c milk

Pepper

1 tsp salt

½ tsp dry mustard

¼ c flour

2 tbsps. butter, divided

4 c cauliflower, steamed

Directions

Once you steam the cauliflower, set it aside. Place three tablespoons of the butter into a pot, allow it to melt and then mix in the seasonings and the flour. Stir in the milk. Mix this until it has thickened up. You should constantly stir to avoid sticking.

Mix in the cheese and pour the mixture over the cauliflower and combine. Sprinkle the bread crumbs if you want to use them and another tablespoon of butter.

Your oven should be set to 375 and place it in and cook for 30 minutes.

This recipe makes a lot of mac and cheese, many servings for bariatric patients as well as the rest of the family. You can also choose to have the recipe as well.

Avocado Tuna Salad

Ingredients

Pepper

Salt

1 lime, juiced

½ red pepper, diced

1 tbsp. pesto

¼ c Greek yogurt, plain

1 can tuna, drained

½ avocado, mashed

Directions

Put all of the above ingredients into a bowl and stir everything together until well mixed. If you are passed the pureed stage, serve with veggies, crackers, or on a sandwich.

Butternut Squash Puree

Ingredients

Pepper

Salt

2 tbsps. coconut oil, butter, or ghee

1 tsp sage, dried – or 1 tbsp. minced sage

1 tbsp. coconut oil or ghee

1 butternut squash

Directions

Your oven should be set at 400 degrees.

Chop up and peel your butternut squash into as even chunks as you can. Coat the squash in the sage and a tablespoon of coconut oil or ghee. Spread the squash out onto a cooking sheet and sprinkle everything with pepper and salt.

Put this in the oven for 30 to 35 minutes, or until the squash has become tender.

Place the roasted squash into a blender, or a food processor if you have one, along with two tablespoons of coconut oil or butter. Mix this up until completely smooth.

Adjust the pepper and salt as you need for your taste.

Street Corn Soup

Ingredients

2 tbsps. + 2 tsp cilantro, divides

1 tsp lime zest

1 tbsp. lime juice

½ c cotija cheese, grated

½ c sour cream

4 c chicken broth

2 garlic cloves, chopped

Pepper

Salt

¼ tsp chili powder

1 c yellow onion, chopped

6 c corn kernels – save 6 cobs for cooking

¼ c olive oil

Directions

Place the oil in a Dutch oven and let it heat up until it begins to shimmer. Place in ½ teaspoon pepper, ½ teaspoon salt, 1/8 teaspoon chili powder, onion, and corn kernels. Cook the mixture, often stirring, until the onions have become soft and the corn begins to brown a little. This should take around ten minutes. Place in the garlic and let cook until it becomes fragrant. Take a cup and a half of this mixture and place it aside. Mix in the broth and the six corn cobs into the Dutch oven. Deglaze the pan to get all the browned bits off the bottom. Allow the mixture to come up to a boil, turn the heat down to a simmer and let it cook for 20 minutes.

Carefully take out the cobs using tongs. Mix in the Cotija and sour cream. Place the mixture, in batches, into a blender and pulse until smooth. You can also use an immersion blender to make it smooth. Place the soup back over the heat. Mix in ¾ of a cup of the reserved corn mixture, two tablespoons of cilantro, and lime juice. Mix in with extra chili powder, pepper, and salt.

Toss the rest of the ¾ cup of reserved corn mixture with two teaspoons of cilantro and lime zest. When serving the soup, add some of the flavored corn mixtures on top and some extra Cotija if you would like.

Banana Custard Pudding

Ingredients

9 bananas, sliced

12 oz. vanilla wafers

1 tsp vanilla extract

¼ c softened butter

4 egg yolks, beaten

7 c milk

¼ c cornstarch

½ c AP flour

2 ½ c sugar

Directions

Mix together the cornstarch, sugar, flour in a bowl.

Place the milk into a big pot and let heat up. You need to bring to 160 F. Slowly add in some of the hot milk into the yolks you beat earlier. Mix the dry ingredients into the tempered eggs and then pour this back into the pot.

As you are constantly stirring, let it cook until it becomes thick and will coat your spoon.

Set the mixture from the heat and mix in the vanilla and butter. Allow the mixture to cool off to room temperature.

Place one-third of your vanilla wafers into the bottom of nine by 13 baking dish. Place half of the banana slices on top of the wafers and then add half of the custard. Top with another third of the wafers, the rest of the bananas and the rest of the custard. Crush up the wafers and sprinkle over the top.

Cauliflower Casserole

Ingredients

Pepper

½ tsp salt

½ c half and half – optional

4 c chicken broth, reduced sodium

2 c water

8 c broccoli, chopped

2 garlic cloves, chopped

1 celery stalk, chopped

1 onion, chopped

1 tbsp. EVOO

1 tbsp. butter

Directions

Place the butter into your Dutch oven and let the butter melt. Mix in the celery and the onion, and cook until they have softened. This will take about four to six minutes. Mix in the thyme and garlic, stirring, until it becomes fragrant.

Mix in the broccoli. Pour in the broth and water and let it come up to a good simmer. Reduce the temp of your heat to maintain the simmer and cook until it is tender. This will take about eight minutes.

In batches, puree your soup in the blender, or use an immersion blender. Mix it back together and add the half and half, if you are using, pepper, and salt.

Egg Custard

Ingredients

Grated nutmeg

2 tsp vanilla

2/3 c Splenda

4 eggs

12 oz. evaporated milk

1 c milk

Directions

Your oven should set your oven to 325. Put six custard cups in a large baking pan and place it to the side.

Place the vanilla, Splenda, eggs, evaporated milk, and milk into your blender and press pulse three to four times until it is well mixed and smooth.

Pour this mixture into the six custard cups evenly. Grate a decent amount of nutmeg over the top of every cup.

Pour hot water into the baking pan so that it comes almost halfway up the custard cup sides. Carefully place this into your oven and cook it for 25 to 35 minutes, or until the center set in the center and still slightly jiggly. Your custards should be set before you take them from the oven.

Carefully take the cups out of the water bath and place a towel to cool off.

Sweet Potato and Beef Puree

Ingredients

1 tbsp. fresh thyme, chopped

2 c beef broth

2 sweet potatoes, chopped and peeled

8 oz. sirloin, cubed

Directions

Place the broth, thyme, sweet potatoes, and beef in a pot and let it all come to a boil. Turn the heat down a bit, so that simmers for 25 to 35 minutes, or until the sweet potatoes are soft and the beef has cooked through. Set this off the heat and allow it to cool a bit.

Place all of this in your blender and mix it up until smooth. Add a little extra broth as needed to thin it out to the consistency that you can eat.

Jell-O Fluff

Ingredients

1 container Greek yogurt, plain

1 c sugar-free Jell-O, set

Directions

Cook your Jell-O according to the box directions and have it completely set before making this recipe. After it has set, measure a cup of it out and place it in the blender with the Greek yogurt. Mix it up until it is smooth. Place in the fridge or the freezer until it has thickened up, and enjoy.

Chicken and Potato Puree

Ingredients

2 c chicken broth

100% Potato Flakes

Directions

Allow the chicken broth to come to a boil. Set it off the heat and stir in the potato flakes, a tablespoon at a time, until your reach pourable texture. If you add too many flakes, just pour in a little more broth. Add pepper and salt to your liking, and enjoy.

Instant Pot Custard

Ingredients

Vanilla, to taste

4 tbsps. Splenda

1 ½ c Fairlife whole milk

3 eggs

1 tbsp. sugar

Directions

Sprinkle a tablespoon of sugar into the bottom of a pot that you can fit in your Instant Pot and set it on the heat until the sugar has melted and become browned. Make sure you don't let this burn.

Place all of the remaining ingredients into your blender and mix it up until smooth and carefully place it in the pot.

Place a cup of water into your Instant Pot and place in the trivet. Place the pot with the custard on to the trivet.

Set your pot to cook for five minutes at high pressure and then let the pressure release naturally.

Once done, set the custard in your refrigerator to cool. After it is cooled, gently unmold it and enjoy.

Taco Casserole

Ingredients

2 c Mexican cheese blend, shredded

1 can tomatoes and chiles

1 can refried beans, fat-free

1 can black beans, rinsed and drained

Envelope taco mix

1 garlic clove, minced

1 small onion, diced

1 small squash, diced

1 small zucchini, diced

1 lb. ground meat, lean

Directions

In a skillet that has been coated with some oil, cook the garlic and veggies until they have become soft. Get rid of any excess liquid that the veggies have created, and then place the veggies in a bowl.

Cook the meat until brown, drain off the grease, and then place it in the bowl with the veggies. Add in the tomatoes and canned black beans and stir it all together.

Sprinkle the mixture with taco seasoning and stir to distribute it. Place the mixture in a casserole dish.

Smooth the refried beans over the mixture. It's easier if you heat up the beans before trying to spread them.

Sprinkle over with the cheese. Your oven should be at 350 and bake it for 30 minutes, or until everything has warmed and the cheese is melted.

Allow the mixture to cool for 20 minutes before your serve it.

Root Beer Float Ice Cream

Ingredients

½ c Diet Root Bee

1 tbsp. vanilla Torani syrup, sugar-free

2 scoops vanilla protein powder

1 c vanilla soy milk

Directions

Place the soda, syrup, protein powder, and milk in a blender or mixer. Mix it up on high until it is lump free and airy. You can also use a milk frother for this to make it really airy. Place this mixture into an ice cream maker and freeze.

You can eat it as is, or you can freeze it to make it a hard ice cream consistency.

St. Patrick's Shake

Ingredients

Ice cubes

1 tbsp. pistachio pudding mix, sugar-free

1 Ready to Drink vanilla protein shake – Premier Protein

Directions

Place all of this into your blender and whizz it up until it is smooth.

Tortilla Soup

Ingredients

½ c corn tortilla strips

1 c Monterey Jack, grated

1 diced avocado

Salt

4 corn tortillas, diced

14 ½ oz. water

2 14.5 oz. can chicken broth

½ tsp cumin

½ tsp minced garlic

½ bunch cilantro, chopped

2 tomatoes, diced

3 tbsps. oil

1 to 2 serrano chili, minced

1 onion, diced

Directions

In your chosen cooking vessel, preferably a large pot, place in three tablespoons of oil, chilies, and onion, and stir-fry this until you see the onions brown along their edges.

Place in the cumin, garlic, cilantro, and tomatoes and stir-fry this for another three to four minutes.

Add in the corn tortillas, water, and broth. The corn tortillas can be diced, or you can tear them up by hand if you want to. Turn the heat up so that the mixture starts to boil. Turn the heat back down to a maintained simmer and let it cook for 10 to 15 minutes. Once done, set this aside so that it can cool down a little bit.

Using a regular blender or an immersion blender, puree up the mixture until it is smooth.

Place this back in the pot and let it heat back up. Check the taste to adjust the salt level.

Garnish the soup with tortilla strips, cheese, and avocado if you desire.

Chicken Broth

Ingredients

Pepper

Thyme sprig

Parsley sprig

Bay leaf

½ celery stalk

½ carrot

½ onion

3 qts water

3 lb. whole chicken

Directions

Grab yourself a large pot and place all of the above in it. Let the mixture come up to a simmer and cook for an hour to an hour and a half. Reserve the cooked chicken for other recipes and strain out and of the other solids.

Place the strained stock in the refrigerator. The following day, skim the fat off that has risen to the top.

Chicken Puree

Ingredients

1 tsp dried parsley

1 c chicken stock

8 oz. chicken thigh or breast, cubed – skinless and boneless

Directions

Place the above ingredients into a pot and let it come up to a boil. Turn the heat down and let it cook for 15 to 20 minutes. The chicken should be cooked all the way through. Allow the mixture to cool for a few minutes.

Place everything in the pot into your blender and mix it up until it is smooth. If you need to, add more stock to get it creamy.

Baked Potato Soup

Ingredients

Pepper

Salt

½ c sour cream

1 ½ c shredded cheese

3 green onions, sliced

6 potatoes, cubed and peeled

4 c milk

14 c AP flour

5 tbsps. butter, unsalted

1 pack bacon, diced

Directions

Place the cubed and peeled potatoes into water and completely cover them with water to keep them from becoming discolored.

Place the diced bacon into a skillet and cook it until crispy and brown. Place this on a paper towel to get rid of any excess grease.

Melt the butter inside of a big pot. Mix in the flour and cook until it has browned up a bit. Slowly whisk in the milk and allow it to cook while you are stirring so that it starts to thicken. Mix in the potatoes and around half of the onions.

Let this boil for a few minutes, and then turn it down and continue to cook until the potatoes are fork tender. This should take about 15 to 20 minutes. Mix in the pepper, sour cream, salt, and cheese. If the soup has become too thick, add in a bit more milk. For the pureed stage use an immersion blender to make the soup smooth.

You can serve it topped with extra cheese, bacon bits, green onions, and sour cream.

Creamy Shrimp Bisque

Ingredients

Pepper

Salt

½ lb. shrimp, deveined and cleaned

1 c evaporated milk, fat-free

1 bottle clam juice

¼ tsp lemon pepper

1 oz. ham, low-fat

1 tsp garlic, chopped

¼ c onion, chopped

Nonstick spray

1 c cauliflower, steamed

Directions

Add some nonstick spray to a large pot and add in the ham, garlic, and onions and let them cook until soft and brown.

Mix in the shrimp, cauliflower, milk, clam juice, and lemon pepper. Allow this mixture to come up to a boil while stirring often. Allow this to continue to cook until the shrimp become pink.

Mix in the pepper and the salt to your taste.

Place the mixture into your blender and mix it up until smooth.

Peanut Brittle Oatmeal

Ingredients

2 tbsps. Torani brown sugar cinnamon syrup, sugar-free

1 tbsp. sweetener, no-calorie

2 tbsps. PB2

Pinch salt

1 scoop vanilla protein powder

½ c quick oats

Directions

Follow the directions for the brand of quick oats you have. Once it is cooked, mix in all of the other above ingredients. Adjust any of the sweeteners that you need to suit your taste buds.

PB2 Shake

Ingredients

½ c ice

1 tbsp. PB2 powder

1 c milk, skim

1 protein powder – chocolate or classic

Directions

Place all of the above ingredients into your blender. Mix it up until smooth or all of the ice has been crushed up and everything how been combined.

Egg Drop Soup

Ingredients

1 c water

1 egg

1 scoop chicken bouillon granules

Directions

Beat the egg in a bowl until well mixed.

Place the water in a pot and heat it up to boiling. Mix in the chicken bouillon until it has dissolved completely.

Take the egg you beat earlier and fork. As you are stirring the water with the fork, slowly add in the egg so that it forms ribbons of cooked egg. Continue until the egg is mixcd in completely. Enjoy.

Yogurt

Ingredients

1 scoop unflavored protein powder

1 c yogurt, favorite fruit flavor – nonfat

Directions

Place all of the above into a bowl and stir together until well mixed. Enjoy.

Sweet Potato Puree

Ingredients

Pepper

Salt

3 large sweet potatoes

Directions

Peel all of the sweet potatoes and then slice them up into two-inch pieces. Place them in a pot and cover them completely with water. Allow the potatoes to boil and cook until they can easily be poked with a fork. This will take about 15 to 20 minutes.

Drain off the water and then puree them in a blender or a food processor if you have one. Mix in some pepper and salt to your taste.

If you want to flavor the sweet potatoes, you can add:

Two tablespoons of maple syrup and butter when you puree the potatoes – Maple Butter

¼ cup of orange juice and milk, two tablespoons of butter, and two teaspoons of ginger when pureeing – Orange Ginger

One tablespoon lime juice and a little bit of cayenne when pureeing – Lime Cayenne

Conclusion

Thank for making it through to the end of *Gastric Bypass Recipes*. Let's hope it was informative and able to provide you with all of the tools you need to achieve your goals.

The next step is to try some of the recipes while you are in your first stages after gastric bypass.

Finally, if you found this book useful in any way, a review on Amazon is always appreciated!

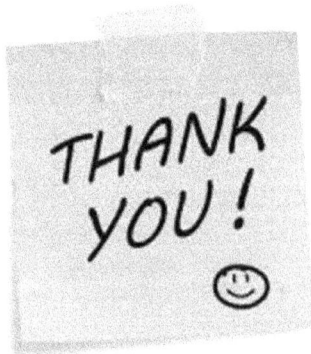

Check Out My Other Books

Below you'll find some of my other popular books that are popular on Amazon and Kindle as well. Simply click on the links below to check them out. Alternatively, you can visit my author page on Amazon to see other work done by me.

CrossFit: Barbell and Dumbbell Exercises for Body Strength

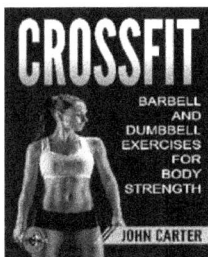

Mediterranean Diet: Step By Step Guide And Proven Recipes For Smart Eating And Weight Loss

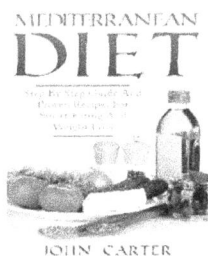

Weight Watchers: Smart Points Cookbook - Step By Step Guide And Proven Recipes For Effective Weight Loss

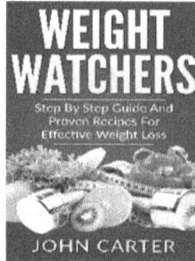

Bodybuilding: Beginners Handbook - Proven Step By Step Guide To Get The Body You Always Dreamed About

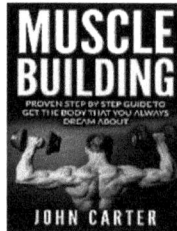

South Beach Diet: Lose Weight and Get Healthy the South Beach Way

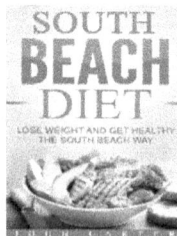

Blood Pressure: Step By Step Guide And Proven Recipes To Lower Your Blood Pressure Without Any Medication

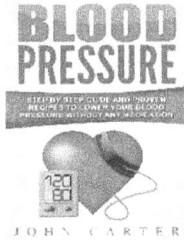

Ketogenic Diet: Step By Step Guide And 70+ Low Carb, Proven Recipes For Rapid Weight Loss

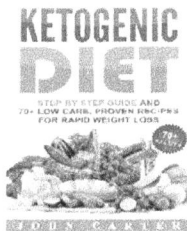

Meal Prep: 65+ Meal Prep Recipes Cookbook – Step By Step Meal Prepping Guide For Rapid Weight Loss

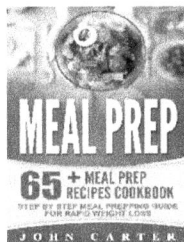

If the links do not work, for whatever reason, you can simply search for these titles on the Amazon website to find them.

www.ingramcontent.com/pod-product-compliance
Lightning Source LLC
Chambersburg PA
CBHW071239020426
42333CB00015B/1543